Do More Eat Less
Best Way to Lose Weight Fast

With Recipes

By: A.E Wilson

Do More Eat Less
Best Way to Lose Weight Fast

With Recipes

By: A.E Wilson

Table of Contents

Introduction

A lot of weight loss books and websites often give out good advice, but oftentimes, no one has the time, money, energy, or the ability to actually do them. In the past years, so many types of diets have come out, each one being touted to be better than other diets. Newfangled exercise equipment, diet shakes and pills are constantly being advertised on TV and in magazines, and too often they seem too good to be true. But in reality, sticking to a mantra made up of four simple words does a lot more for weight loss and fitness than any kind of weight loss pill will ever do.

Do More, Eat Less.
In this book, myths on exercise and dieting will be debunked. With so many experts pushing the latest and best techniques to achieve weight loss, sometimes, the search for what really works lead to a lot of myths and misleading information. In this chapter, you'll learn if drinking lots of water will really lead to weight loss, if vegetarian diets are better than meat inclusive ones, and if carbohydrates are bad for you. You'll also learn if there are any truths to exercise myths. Will doing crunches and ab workouts really get rid of belly fat? Should women never lift weights? Here, you'll find out what really works, and what doesn't when it comes to slimming down.

You'll also learn about changing the way you workout. Because exercise is definitely a priority when it comes to staying healthy, it doesn't need to be done exclusively to lose weight. Working out has many physical and mental health benefits, and if you don't fancy going to a gym to sweat it out among strangers, there are other things that you can do to get inspired to start exercising, which you'll know all about in this book.

Exercise is a must throughout one's life, and it's very important to stay active even through your senior years. Though getting older brings on a host of things that impairs mobility, this shouldn't discourage you from working out. Studies show that staying active may benefit you by making you stronger, more flexible, and it helps older adults maintain and lose weight. Find out how to work out safely and effectively during your senior years.

Aside from sticking to an exercise regimen, changing the way you eat is also key to achieving weight loss. Healthy eating does not mean depriving yourself of the foods you love or staying unrealistically thin, but about developing a well-balanced and satisfying relationship with food. Your food choices will not only make you slim, but will reduce your risk of illnesses such as heart disease, cancer, and diabetes. Learn about making small but powerful changes that you can do that can result to lasting weight loss.

Lastly, learn about all kinds of healthy recipes that are not only delicious, but are truly good for you. Soup and stew recipes that can fill you up and warm you can contribute to weight loss and your overall health. Salads that incorporate fruits and vegetables without the addition of fattening dressings can be a valuable addition to your everyday meals. And healthy snacks can help you regulate your blood sugar levels and help you avoid overeating at your next meal.

Indeed, the simplest ways to being healthy and losing weight are the ones that work best. Do More, Eat Less!

By: E. A Wilson

Chapter 1: Myths on Exercise and Diet

A common indicator of being in the pink of health is being in shape. It's easily said than done though, as many often resort to extreme measures for this to happen. People have different motivations for maintaining a healthy weight—it could be to maintain good blood pressure, lower the risks of obesity-related diseases such as hypertension and diabetes, or simply, to look and feel great. And with all these motivators, a lot of individuals will turn to the tried and true methods to achieve weight loss. These methods are diet, and exercise.

With so many experts pushing the latest and best techniques to achieve weight loss, sometimes, the search for what really works lead to a lot of myths. Here are the most popular myths in fitness and diet:

Diet Myths

1. Drinking water can help you lose weight.
Consuming copious amounts of water is often touted to be the best way to lose weight. This is not true. It's also not true that drinking more water will cause you to feel full, and thus will make you eat less solid food. Water should be consumed to keep the body hydrated, and it can flush toxins out of your system, but when it comes to weight loss, sorry to say, but it really doesn't help at all.

2. Vegetarian diets are healthier and lower in calories than meat inclusive ones.
Eating lots of veggies is healthy. But cutting out an entire food group is not such a good idea. Meat is a key source of iron, which keeps energy levels up. It allows you to think clearly, and meat produces enzymes that fight infection. Moreover, studies have shown that an iron deficiency increases the risk for women to develop postpartum depression. Though vegetarians get their iron from lentils, cereals, tofu and beans, it's not enough to provide the required amount of protein that a body should get. If you're a vegetarian, make sure to eat eggs, dairy products or soy at every meal to get your required dose of protein

3. To avoid gaining weight, you shouldn't eat late at night.
Calories can't tell time. Our bodies process calories in the same way, no matter what time we eat our meals. This myth comes from the choices we make for late night snacking—processed foods, or foods high in fat or extra sugars. It's better to avoid bingeing on these types of food and have a healthy snack instead.

4. Carbs are bad for you.

Carbohydrates don't make you fat, but extra calories do. Moderation is the key when it comes to consuming any kind of food. Carbohydrates are found not only in bread or pasta, it can also be found in fruits, vegetables, and whole grains. It's an important addition to any diet, so don't rule out carbs. The trick is to lessen the consumption of simple carbs, and to choose more complex carbs.

5. Diet foods will help you lose weight.

Words or labels that say low fat or low sugar doesn't necessarily mean low calorie. Foods that are sold in the market as diet foods are loaded with hidden dangers such as artificial sweeteners and preservatives. If ever you are tempted to try the diet version of your favorite food, keep in mind that it's better to have a small portion of the real thing rather than bingeing on the diet food. It will taste better, and it will keep cravings at bay.

6. If you're eating healthfully, you can eat as much as you want.

A calorie is a calorie, no matter where it comes from. While it's true that it's healthier for you to eat only nutritious food, eating too much of anything will still cause you to pack on the pounds.

7. Fat and oils will make you fat.

Yes, fat does contain more calories than protein or carbs, but that doesn't mean that you should shun it altogether from your diet. When eaten in moderation, fat will not only help you feel fuller, it also helps your body to absorb certain vitamins and phytonutrients, which will lead to a healthier you.

8. **The only way to lose weight is to drastically cut down on calories.**

Sure, if you dramatically reduce the amount of calories that you take in, you're sure to see equally dramatic results within weeks, but this weight loss won't be the long term kind. Not only is this type of dieting nearly impossible to sustain, it's unhealthy and can cause serious repercussions to your health. Many people who have tried extreme diets have found out that they gain back the weight they've lost, and even gain some additional pounds once they stop. Once the body is starved, it hoards calories because it doesn't know when it will get fed again. This is the reason why so many people gain more weight after stopping the diet.

9. **Skipping meals is a good way to lose weight**

In theory, skipping a meal while keeping everything else in your diet the same will help you lose weight. But whenever you skip a meal, your eating pattern changes. There's a tendency to overeat and overcompensate later, which will inevitably lead to weight gain.

Exercise Myths

1. Women should never lift weights because it will make them bulky.
It's actually very difficult to create bulk, and women's bodies have too much estrogen to create large muscles. For men, it's easier to bulk up because they have testosterone. Because muscle takes up less space than fat, strength training will actually make muscles appear shapelier, not bigger. Women should lift weights once in a while to decrease body fat, increase lean muscle mass, and burn calories more efficiently.

2. Low-intensity exercise burns more fat.
In general, low-intensity workouts may be ideal for most people as it's less stressful on the joints. But the truth is, the more intensely you exercise, the higher proportion of carbs you'll burn. When the body has burned up all the carbs, it starts burning fat.

3. If you go to the gym and workout for 30 to 45 minutes a day, that gives you a free pass to do or eat whatever you want for the rest of the day.
Going to the gym doesn't negate a bad diet or unhealthy habits. Studies have shown that if you're sedentary most of the day, then it doesn't matter how hard or how often you exercise. Ditto if you scarf a few fast food treats after working out.

4. The more you work out, the better.

While it's recommended for the average healthy adult to work out for at least 150 minutes per week, working out more than this or performing the same activity each day can have a negative effect on one's health. Joints and muscles need a break to repair themselves, and overworking them will leave you prone to injuries.

5. Doing crunches and ab workouts will get rid of belly fat.

No amount of crunches will give you a 6-pack stomach, because if you have a high percentage of body fat, then your abs will be covered with fat. Doing ab exercises won't make you lose that belly fat either. You can't spot-train, and the only way to get visibly toned abs is to reduce the overall body fat first, which means plenty of cardio coupled with strength training.

Chapter 2: Changing the Way You Workout

Every year, Americans spend an average of $60 billion on gym memberships to lose weight, with each membership costing about $50 in average. But there are some who would rather not spend the money on exercise, instead, they focus on eating organic food, taking supplements and vitamins, and going on spa retreats and juice cleanses, thinking that by doing these things, the pounds will just melt right off.

Though there's nothing wrong with eating healthfully and taking vitamins, doing these things alone will not guarantee weight loss. And spa retreats and juice cleanses, when done regularly, will result to immediate weight loss, but the effects are temporary at best. Studies have also shown that depriving the body of essential nutrients coupled by lack of exercise can lead to health problems later in life.

Exercise should definitely be a priority when it comes to being healthy, and no, it doesn't necessarily have to be done to lose weight. Even a person who is currently at his or her ideal weight should exercise and get moving to enjoy the full health benefits of having an active lifestyle.

A lot of people hit the gym or pound the pavement to build muscle, improve cardiovascular health and get an improved physique, but working out has other benefits. For the past years, scientists have studied how exercising can boost brain function. Regardless of age or fitness level, studies show that making time for exercise provides a lot of health benefits.

Exercise helps reduce stress. If you've had a rough day at the office, you can take a walk or head to the gym for a quick workout. Working up a sweat helps manage physical and mental stress. When you exercise, you increase your brain's production of the chemical called norepinephrine, which helps the brain respond better to stress.

Working out can also boost endorphins, which create feelings of happiness and euphoria. Studies have shown that exercise can alleviate symptoms among the clinically depressed, and for this reason, doctors recommend that those who are suffering from anxiety or depression should take the time to get some exercise. Working out for just 30 minutes a few times a week can do wonders to boost your overall mood.

Everyone has an activity or form of exercise that will best suit his age, capability, and at the same time keep one engaged and motivated to keep on doing it. Ask yourself the following questions before committing to an exercise program:

- Do you like to work out alone or with a group?
- Would you prefer to exercise in a gym or outdoors?
- Does routine bore you? Would you like to have more variety in your workouts?
- How much time can you honestly give yourself to exercise, and how many days a week can you commit to it?
- Are you athletic? Have you participated in a sport when you were younger, and if given the chance, would you like to do it again?
- Can you exercise independently, or do you need to work with a coach or personal trainer?

Once you answer these questions, you'll be able to find out the type of physical activity that's right for you. Don't feel pressured into taking a class or enrolling in a gym if that doesn't feel right for you. You'll be better off doing an activity that you love, because you're more likely to stick with it in the long run.

Here are the types of activities that you can do, based on your fitness personality:

1. If you like working out with a group, and if you are athletic, and you have an innate competitive nature, then you could:

a. **Join your community baseball, basketball, ice hockey, soccer or other sports team.**

Relive your childhood days and join a sports team. Not only is it a great way to make friends, but you get to enjoy playing with a team, and get into the competitive nature of the sport while keeping the pounds at bay. If your neighborhood does not have an existing team, round up a group of friends who would love to play the same sport as you. You might have to invest in the necessary equipment for the sport if you plan on doing this regularly, so that'll mean some comfortable basketball shorts and sneakers for basketball, cleats for soccer, a helmet and protective equipment and a hockey stick for ice hockey, and so on.

Martial arts would also be a good fit for you. Not only do you get trained to protect yourself if you need to do so, but this enhances your ability to focus and it also makes you more agile and strong. You will need to be properly attired for this, so ask your instructor for guidance on what to wear.

2. If you have a natural sense of rhythm, are graceful, easily bored with routine and love to work out with a group:

Check out a yoga or a dance class

If you like going out with friends to go dancing, then this could be the right fit for you. What better way to sweat off the weight than with an energy-filled dance class? Dancing is a fun way to keep fit. It improves your coordination and flexibility and as an added bonus, you can bust out the moves you learned in class when you attend parties or go out dancing with friends. All you need are some running shoes with good traction (you don't even need shoes with fancy brands, just pick ones that are comfortable and won't make you slip and slide all over the place), sweat pants and cotton shirts that skim the body (nothing too baggy, since you can't check your form that way), a membership to a dance class and some good dance music, and you're all good to go. If you can't afford to join a class, you can do this at home. There are online videos that you can look up to get your dance on for free. Youtube is a great resource for this. You can go on different channels and try them out to find the style that suits you best. Some notable Youtube channels are:

- BeFIT- this is an exercise channel from Lionsgate which offers new workouts every single weekday. Trainers include Jillian Michaels, Denise Austin and Jane Fonda, among others.
- SparkPeople Videos- this channel has playlists for pregnancy workouts, swimsuit boot camps, and more.

You could also buy fitness DVDs. If you want to move on to more advanced dance moves and choreography, here are the best DVDs that you can buy:

- Paula Abdul's Get Up and Dance!- it will take you back to the 80's! For a bit of nostalgia and some great coaching from Paula herself, this workout video is it.
- Tribal Energy Cardio- This hour-long video adapts Western African dance movements into a total body workout that is fun and makes you feel really good.
- Hemalayaa's The Bollywood Dance Workout- Almost an hour of Bollywood-style movements, mixed with hip-hop, belly-dance, Indian, classical and Bhangra dance moves.
- Billy Blanks Jr.'s Dance With Me Groove and Burn- This DVD has a variety of dance styles and fun tunes.

Yoga, on the other hand, keeps you centered and makes you increasingly strong and flexible as you go on day by day. Many celebrities such as Madonna, Jennifer Aniston and Gwyneth Paltrow are hooked on yoga, and as you can see, they have long and lean muscles from holding all the yoga poses. For equipment, you'll only need a yoga mat (make sure it's non-skid to prevent accidents), and some yoga pants, and a top that won't flop over your head when you do inversions.

You can also do yoga at home. Here are some great Youtube channels for free yoga sessions:

- Blogilates- Instructor Cassey Ho offers a lighthearted and lively approach to yoga and fitness instruction, ideal for a younger audience.
- Yogasync.TV- this Youtube channel boasts a huge library of guided yoga lessons that you can do for 20 minutes. If you stick to the session and do this at least three times a week, you'll find yourself doing much more complicated poses in a matter of weeks.

If you're on the lookout for a good yoga DVD, consider these selections.

- Yoga Journal Complete Beginner's Guide- A lot of yoga DVDs claim to be for beginners, but they need some familiarity with yoga poses which makes them totally inappropriate for true beginners. If you've never done yoga, this is the workout video for you.
- Yogalosophy- Celebrity trainer Mandy Ingber (Jennifer Aniston is her best client) incorporates dynamic toning exercises to traditional yoga poses.

3. If you like to work out alone, have never exercised before, but you're willing to put in the time and effort:

By: E. A Wilson

Try running, swimming, or working out in a gym with a personal trainer

If you've never exercised before and are anxious to get results, the best thing that you could do is to work out in a gym with a personal trainer. A personal trainer will motivate you and guide you to make sure that you get the body that you want. Just like athletes have their coaches, your trainer will look out for your best interests when it comes to meeting your fitness goals. The best trainers are the ones who can deliver results in the least amount of time as possible. Ask for referrals from people who have lost weight with the help from their trainer. Find a trainer that can serve as a fitness role model, has good credentials, and has a personality that you like. So many people have skipped out on workouts because they dread their trainers, which is a shame because these people pay their trainers to motivate them, not humiliate or bully them. A good trainer must be able to motivate in a positive manner as well as offer constructive criticism when necessary. Some people might like the strict, military style approach, while others might do better with someone who has a gentler manner. Pick a trainer who you'll be comfortable working out with so that you'll look forward to your sessions instead of finding ways to avoid them like the plague. Keep in mind that the gym fee will cost you about $50 per month, and on top of that you'll have to pay the trainer fee which is about $50 per session. You'll also need to wear athletic shoes, and some supportive underwear.

If you dislike the feeling of being cooped up in a gym, you can always take up running. It's free and all you'll need is a good pair of running shoes. It can be done anytime, anywhere, it will increase your stamina and it's a good cardio workout. You can do running solely, or do it in addition to other workouts such as strength training. Plan on gradually increasing distances as you progress, or maybe picking up the speed every now and then to see how fast you can go. You can also do this in preparation to joining marathons, which can be really rewarding once you complete them.

If you want something more low impact, try speed walking. This is kinder to the joints and muscles than running, and is a good activity for older adults. Wear some headphones while speed-walking in the park so you can have good music to exercise to, and you can also plan on inviting your family and friends to workout with you.

Swimming is another activity that is low impact and suited to those who live near the water. If you live near the beach or if you have access to a pool, and you're not opposed to getting wet, then this workout is for you. A bathing suit, a swimming cap and some goggles are all you'll need for this. Swimming will give you a lean body and it's something that you can do alone or with family and friends.

There are so many ways to get fit, it's just a matter of finding out what works for you and your budget. Once you find the right workout for you, you'll look forward to doing it, and you'll be fitter and healthier.

Chapter 3: What's Hot and Trendy in Exercise Right Now

If you're bored with running, or with your daily routine at the gym, why not check out the latest trends in exercise? Fitness experts say that this year, workouts will become shorter, getting stronger is done the smart way, and individual goals are the biggest target. This is certainly good news for many people who are finding it harder and harder to make the time to exercise. Among the top excuses for not exercising are:

- Lack of time
- Lack of budget
- Boredom with routine
- Having no idea what to do

All the featured work outs in this chapter will solve all your workout woes, and soon you might be running out of excuses why you can't workout. Some of these workouts even cost less than the average amount it takes to work out at the gym with a personal trainer.

1. **Fusion Fitness**

Fusion fitness will take this year by storm as people work to burn as many calories as possible in a short amount of time. If you only have an hour to work out, then this could be a good fit for you. The key to good results is to combine strength training, cardio and flexibility training into one workout, increasing repetitions with low weight to keep heart rate up during the entire session. It's definitely not about lifting heavy weights, as doing Fusion Fitness while lifting more than 8 pounds over the head is not recommended.

2. **Stability Training**

Stability Training builds strength throughout the body while helping to prevent injury. Concentrating on your form while you exercise can help you become stronger by using your body's current state of resistance. It's good to work stability training along with balancing exercises that uses your body weight.

3. **Weighted Hula Hoop**

A favorite of those who grew up playing with this old-school toy, and it has become incorporated into a lot of women's fitness routine, most especially senior citizens. Using a weighted hula hoop will tone your thighs, abs, glutes, and arms—and burn about 200 calories in 30 minutes. You can crank up your favorite music and start hula hooping, even in your own backyard.

4. Pole Workouts

Whatever you may feel about the explosion of the pole dance industry in recent years, classes in the highly athletic dance form have, in fact become all the rage for women who want an acrobatic, fun workout that strengthens and tones. The women-only classes combine dance moves with pole tricks involving suspension and stretching—the dance portion gets the heart rate up as a cardio workout, while doing tricks on the pole strengthens your upper and lower body, especially your core.

5. Indoor surfing

Using the RipSurferX, the world's first total body surf trainer designed to mimic real surfing, one can absolutely get fit while balancing, just without the ocean. The board has bands on either side of it that controls how much it teeters, and most of the top of the board is covered with black matting. You use your core to mimic real surfing movements and then mix them with cardio bursts to burn fat. You'll improve balance, define muscles, and best of all, you won't even need sunblock.

6. Aerial Yoga

If you're ready to find a new yoga challenge, it might be time to get up in the air. Aerial yoga adapts traditional yoga moves while in a large silk hammock that's suspended off the ground. The instructor will teach you to twist and maneuver your way into stretches while working your core and relieving stress.

7. **Street Boing**

If you don't mind looking a bit silly while you work out, then try Street Boing. You'll be using Kangoo Jump shoes to spice up your workout that is guaranteed to be lots of fun. The queer looking shoes actually add gravitational force to your body, thus doubling the resistance of your aerobics while wearing them. The shoes were originally designed as a way to relieve the stress on runners' joints, and they reduce joint stress while still making you work up a sweat. Some gyms have street boing classes strictly indoors, while other gyms will have you graduate to pounding the pavement while perform sports drills, sprints and plyometrics exercises.

8. **Barre**

If you ever wanted a ballerina's body—long, defined muscles, tight stomach and buttocks, and an allover lean look, then you're in luck. Barre workouts will get you looking like your favorite prima ballerina in no time. The ballet inspired moves use yoga, Pilates, and weight training to lengthen muscles and reshape your entire body. While you're using your entire body, your legs will especially feel the burn.

9. **Fencing**

Sword fighting is once again in vogue, thanks in part to many Game of Thrones fans. If you want an activity that will work your mind as well as your body, it's time to take up fencing. Essentially, this is sword fighting but without the risk of losing limbs. Fencing forces you to make fast, accurate decisions while dueling. This fast-paced workout will raise your heart rate while improving speed, agility, hone your reflexes, and will tone your muscles.

10. **Mini Trampolines**

Mini trampolines known as rebounders are taking fitness gyms by storm. Trampolines provide an intensive workout that you can do at home or at the gym. They're a fun way to get your cardio in without it feeling like a chore. Keeping steady while doing your moves will tighten your abs and improve leg power and strength, without increasing pressure on your joints, making this a wonderful low-impact workout.

11. **Ultimate Frisbee**

Are you naturally competitive, likes playing in a team, and hates to be cooped up indoors while exercising? The Ultimate Frisbee workout will be a great fit for you. It's an intense game, and without referees, it's rooted in sportsmanship and team play. While you're having fun with your buddies, you'll be burning calories as you run and pass the Frisbee to your teammates across the length of a soccer game.

12. **Salsa Dancing**

It doesn't matter if you're the first one on the dance floor, or if you're an uncoordinated wallflower. Salsa dancing has something to offer everyone. The seductive dance is cardio-heavy, and an hour of dancing will burn about 600 calories. The more you practice, the more confident you'll get, and the smoother your moves will be. You'll be absolutely scintillating the next time you hit the dance floor. If you're looking forward to doing something with your partner, try this, as this is a great workout for couples. And if you're single, well, who knows, you might even find your perfect partner here.

13. Cycle Karaoke

You've gone biking, sure. And you certainly have tried karaoke with your friends. But have you ever tried doing both activities at the same time? Is it a bit weird? Maybe. Is it fun? Absolutely! In this class, you'll be singing, grooving and moving while working up a sweat. It could be the most fun that you could have on a bike, so leave your inhibitions at home and get ready to belt out some tunes.

14. Street Fighter

Ever wish that you could do the cool moves you see on action movies? Whether it's the moves of Cameron Diaz in Charlie's Angels, or Keanu Reeves' action sequences in the Matrix Trilogies that have you wishing that you could look just as cool, then try the Street Fighter workout. You can improve your strength and agility with a combination of martial arts, dance and basic gymnastics moves.

15. Tabura

Tabura is a Swahili name for training used to improve endurance and strength in Africa's military. This fun class uses kickboxing combinations and basic West African dance moves set to Tribal House music and a live drummer. If you're so over your belly dancing class, give this work out a shot.

Chapter 4: Staying Active During Your Senior Years

As you grow older, you'll find that sometimes, it's really hard to maintain an active lifestyle. Getting older brings on a host of things that impairs mobility—you become less flexible, bones start to become more brittle, and joints sometimes feel painful. But these shouldn't stop you from working out. During your senior years, an active lifestyle is more important than ever. Regular exercise can boost energy, manage symptoms of illness or pain, and maintain your independence. In fact, exercise can even reverse some of the symptoms of aging, such as arthritis. Studies show that light intensity activity everyday may reduce the chance of disability in adults with, or at risk of developing knee arthritis. Not only is exercise good for your body, it's good for your mind, memory, and general mood. Whether you are perfectly healthy or managing an illness, there are plenty of ways to stay active during your senior years.

Starting an exercise routine can be a challenge sometimes, especially when you're older. You may feel hampered by illness, ongoing health problems, or fear of injuries or falls. If this is your first time to exercise, you may not have an idea where to begin. Or perhaps you might feel that exercise is simply not for you.

Though all of these may seem good enough reasons to take it easy, there are more reasons why you should start to get moving. Working out can relieve stress, help you manage symptoms of pain or illness, and improve your sense of well-being. Exercise is the key to staying strong and healthy, and it can be fun too!

Here are the benefits of exercising:

- It helps you look and feel younger and stay active longer. Regular physical activity lowers your risk for several conditions, including Alzheimer's, dementia, diabetes, heart disease, high blood pressure, obesity, and colon cancer.
- Studies show that a sedentary lifestyle is unhealthy for adults over 50. Inactivity causes older adults to lose the ability to do things on their own and can lead to hospitalizations. The more you exercise, the longer you stay independent, and the more you save on healthcare costs.
- It builds strength and stamina, prevents loss of bone mass and improves balance, thus lessening the risks of falling.
- Even those who are wheelchair-bound can lift weights, stretch and do chair aerobics to improve muscle tone, range of motion, and promote cardiovascular health.
- It can help older adults maintain and lose weight. As metabolism slows with age, maintaining a healthy weight can be quite a challenge. Exercise can increase metabolism and builds muscle mass, and helps burn more calories. Once you reach a healthy weight, you'll feel better, and your overall health will be greatly improved.
- It reduces the impact of illness and chronic disease. Once you exercise regularly, you'll find that your blood pressure will become lower, you'll have better heart health and bone density, and even better digestive functioning.

- It helps you sleep better. Poor sleep is one of the inevitable consequences of getting older, but this can be remedied by exercise, as it helps you fall asleep more quickly and sleep deeply.
- Endorphins produced by exercise can make you feel better and reduce feelings of sadness or depression. It also increases your confidence and helps you feel sure of yourself.

Committing to a routine of regular physical activity could be one of the best things that you could do to improve your health. Now, a couple of things before you start exercising, just to be safe:

1. Get a medical clearance from your doctor before starting any exercise program, especially if you have a preexisting condition. Be sure to ask if there are any activities that you should avoid doing.

2. Start slo

w. If it's been a while since you've been very active, then it could be harmful if you go all out once you decide to start exercising again. Build up your exercise routine little by little, starting with some low impact activities to start with like stretching or walking. Try just one class a week and see what feels right for you. If you don't feel like joining a class, you can exercise on your own, but make sure to start slowly but surely. Maybe today, you can walk for about two blocks, then the next day try going for three blocks, and so on.

3. Consider your health concerns. Always keep in mind how your current health condition affects your workouts. For instance, if you have diabetes, you may have to adjust the timing of medication and meal plans when making an exercise schedule. If during workouts, something does not feel right, such as you get a sudden sharp, or shortness of breath, then stop. You might need to scale back or try another activity.

4. Commit to an exercise schedule for at least 3 to 4 weeks so that it becomes a habit, and it also takes that long before you start seeing results.
5. Focus on short-term goals to stay motivated, such as improving your energy levels and reducing stress, rather than long-term goals such as weight loss which can take several weeks to achieve.

6. Exercise should never hurt nor make you feel worse than when you first started doing it. Stop exercising immediately and call your doctor if your feel dizzy or short of breath, develop a chest pain or if your blood pressure increases, or if you experience pain. Now that that's out of the way, this is when you start thinking about the activities that you could do. For a balanced exercise plan, you should mix different types of exercises to improve your health and keep you motivated. There are four building blocks for senior fitness, and they are: cardio endurance exercise, strength and power training, flexibility, and balance. There are different activities to fulfill each fitness building block. The key is to find activities that you enjoy doing.

Cardio endurance workouts can help keep your heart pumping and you may feel a bit short of breath. Cardio workouts include

- walking,
- climbing stairs
- swimming
- cycling
- hiking
- tennis
- rowing
- dancing.

These workouts are all good for you as they help lessen fatigue. They also promote independence by improving endurance. Keep in mind that other activities, such as house cleaning or going on errands are also forms of cardio workouts.

Strength building exercises builds muscle through repetitive motion using weight or external resistance from body weight, free weights, machines or elastic bands. Historically, strength training was limited to athletes, but in the past two decades, its popularity has spread to the general public. During a strength workout, the heart's muscle tissue contracts forcefully to push the blood out. This causes small tears in the muscle fibers, and when the body repairs those tears, the heart gets stronger, not just one that is efficient at pumping. Working out with weights also improves glucose metabolism, which can reduce the risk of diabetes. Hence, it's important to build up one's strength to build muscle, prevent loss of bone mass, improve balance, have a stronger heart and lower overall glucose levels. All of these are important so one could stay active and avoid falls. Building strength helps you do ordinary day to day activities such as lifting objects or opening jars.

To improve flexibility, you can do stationary stretches and stretches that involve movement to keep your muscles and joints supple, thus less prone to injury. Studies have shown that stretching relieves arthritis, even more so than type of exercise. Stretching helps your body stay limber by increasing your range of movement for ordinary activities like driving, tying your shoes, washing your hair, or playing with your grandchildren.

Lastly, maintaining balance is important whether you're stationary or moving around. As we get older, our sense of balance may be affected due to several factors, such as blurring of vision, spinal degeneration, and even some medications can cause us to become a bit dizzy and lose our balance. To improve your balance, you can do some exercises such as standing on one foot, walking heel to toe, and doing back leg and side leg raises. Do these exercises slowly, and make sure that you have something beside you to hold on to—such as a chair--if you begin to wobble.

If you dread working out, there are so many ways that you can incorporate the things you enjoy doing into an exercise routine, such as:

- Chatting with a friend or your partner while walking or stretching
- Window shopping while walking around the mall
- Taking photographs while hiking
- Watching your favorite movie while you're on the treadmill

Being active doesn't also need to be limited to working out. Simply changing the way you do regular activities can help you be more active throughout the day, like:

- choosing stairs over elevators, especially if your floor is just on the second or third floor of the building
- parking at the far end of the parking lot when arriving at appointments
- walking down every aisle of the grocery store while shopping
- doing a set of wall push-ups while waiting for your food to finish cooking

- lifting light weights while watching the news
- doing knee bends while talking on the phone

The best thing about working out is that it gives you more energy for activities, which will make you and your loved ones happy. When working out becomes a habit, you'll never want to give it up.

Chapter 5: Getting Started to Work Out

If you're not ready to commit to a structured exercise program or if you don't know how to get started, don't worry. Many people have felt the same way as you, with some feeling a bit embarrassed as they attempt to halfheartedly jog around the block. Some people fail to start or commit to working out because they have doubts if they will really work, and some aren't sure about their level of motivation to stick to it all throughout. And there are some people who had some bad experiences with former personal trainers that it has turned them off from working out ever again.

It seems as if every time you attempt to start an ambitious workout program with the goal of getting in shape, something—you're not even sure what—cuts you short before you've reached your goal. Deep down though, you know what the problem is: you don't like working out. It's uncomfortable, it's sweaty, and some of the gyms you've been to have a weird smell. Plus, you don't even like how you look in those hideous workout clothes, and you're not even sure if you have the time to do it.

Believe it or not, exercising doesn't have to be unpleasant. Don't let all these reasons stop you from being healthy and strong to do more of the things that you would like to do. Wouldn't it be great if you could walk for longer distances without getting short of breath? Or shop and try on clothes that you wouldn't normally get, but now you could because you're in much better shape? And wouldn't it be nice to play a game with your child or grandchild and not feel winded? These are just some reasons why you should start exercising, and one thing that should help you start is to change the way you think about physical activity.

When you've been living a sedentary lifestyle for a long time and then start thinking about working out, any exercise regimen might appear to be quite overwhelming. The key here is to think about physical activity as a lifestyle choice rather than a single task to check off your to-do list. Look at your daily routine and consider ways to sneak in activity here and there. Even small activities can add up over the course of the day to burn off calories.

For instance, here are some things that you could do while you're at home, out and about, or with your family and friends:

In and around your home
- Clean the house
- Wash your car
- Tend to the yard and garden
- Mow the lawn with a push mower rather than using a motor-powered one
- Sweep the sidewalk or patio with a broom
- Rake the leaves instead of having the kids do it.

At work and out and about
- Look for ways to walk or cycle more. For example, you can walk to an appointment rather than drive, especially if it is just a few blocks away from your home.
- Banish elevators and use the stairs. If your appointment is just on the second or third floor, consider using the stairs.
- Walk briskly to the bus stop, then get off one stop early.
- Park at the back of the lot then walk to the store or office

- Take a vigorous walk during your coffee break
- Get up and walk while talking on your cell phone.

With friends and family

- Jog or walk around the soccer field during your kid's practice
- Make a neighborhood bike ride part of your weekend routine
- Play tag with your children in the yard
- Walk the dog together as a family
- If you don't have your own dog, volunteer to walk a dog from the shelter
- Organize an office bowling team
- Take a dance class with your partner or sibling

Exercise doesn't need to be an all or nothing commitment. If you have not exercised before or you've tried an exercise program in the past and been unable to stick with, it's important not to set unrealistic goals. If you're just starting to have a more active lifestyle, then your goal shouldn't be to get buff or lose weight. The first step is to get to that level when you no longer hate to exercise. And then, once you're feeling better about all that physical activity, then you'll have a better chance of sticking to a workout program, and it will also be easier for you to find an exercise routine that you'll love.

When you first start your program, don't force yourself to do anything hard or unpleasant. Start with simple things that you can do regularly, such as stretching. Studies have shown that stretching is more beneficial to relieve arthritis, even more so than exercise. It's also important to stretch before and after exercising, because forgetting to do so will result in stiff and pulled muscles. If you combine stretching with some weight bearing movements, you'll get the best results.

To do this, start by warming up with slow movements, such as head rotations, followed by shoulder rotations, then stretch out your arms and slowly make slow circles with your outstretched arms. Do 8 counts for two repetitions with each movement. Then continue on to hip rotations, and after that march in place. Now you're ready to do some stretching.

Remember to stretch gently, and don't bounce while doing so. If you feel pain, then you've stretched too far. Here's a simple stretching routine that you can do. Make sure to hold each stretch for 15-30 seconds, repeating two or three times, depending on how you feel.

- Neck Stretch- Sit or stand with shoulders relaxed, back straight. Bring your left ear down to your left shoulder and hold. Roll your head down toward the ground and bring your chin to your chest. Hold, then roll your head to the right and bring your right ear to your right shoulder. Inhale and exhale in a slow and controlled manner.

- Hamstring Stretch- Stand tall with your back straight, abs engaged, shoulders down, and feet hip-width apart. Bring your left leg forward, heel down, toes up and leg straight. Keeping your back straight and your abs engaged, bend the right knee as if sitting back, while supporting yourself with both hands on your thighs. Repeat on opposite side.

- Quad Stretch- Stand tall, and hold on to a chair for balance. Keep your feet hip-width apart and your back straight, and your feet parallel. Reach back and grab your left foot with your left hand, keeping your thighs lined up next to each other and left leg in line with the hip. Repeat on opposite side.

- Chest and Biceps Stretch- Stand tall or sit upright. Interlace your fingers behind your back and straighten your arms. With arms straight, lift your arms up behind you while keeping your back straight and your shoulders down. Keep the shoulders down.

- Standing Triceps Stretch- Stand tall. Place your left elbow in your right hand. Reach your left arm overhead, placing palm on the center of your back while supporting your elbow in your right hand. Reach your fingertips down your spine. Keep your shoulders relaxed. Repeat with opposite arm.

Now you can start your workout slowly, then gradually pick up the pace. Give yourself time to slow down during the last 15 minutes of your workout. Don't just stop suddenly and sit down. You have to allow your heart rate to adjust, then finish off with some gentle stretching. Take a moment to relax after you workout, and resist the urge to rush off to do something immediately after you work out.

As for finding the right workout for you, you can focus on activities that you enjoy. For instance, if you hate running, you won't be able to maintain a running program, but if you love swimming or dancing, you'll find it easier to stick with an exercise program that's built around those activities.

Take it slow. Start with an activity you feel comfortable doing, go at your own pace, and keep your expectations realistic.

Focus on short term goals such as improving your mood and energy levels, rather than aiming to reduce weight or build muscle

Make exercise a priority. If you're having trouble fitting in exercise into your schedule, consider it an important appointment with yourself and mark it on your calendar. Commit to exercise at least 3 to 4 days a week so that it becomes habit, and force yourself to stick to it. Even the busiest among us can find a 10-minute slot in a day to take a walk around the block or walk up a single flight of stairs.

Go easy on yourself. Instead of being your worst critic, try a new way to think about your body. No matter what your weight, age, or fitness level, there are certainly others like you with the same goals and reasons for exercising. Try to surround yourself with people who have the same goals. Remember, accomplishing even the smallest fitness goals will help you gain confidence.

Be consistent. Make your workouts habitual by exercising at the same time every day, if possible. Eventually, you'll get to the point where you feel better every time you exercise, and that's a strong incentive to get up and get moving.

Try to keep an exercise journal to record your progress. In a few months, it will be fun to look back on when and how you began. It also holds you accountable to your routine.

Another way to keep you motivated and inspire you to carry on is to talk to your family and colleagues about your fitness routines. You might be surprised to find out that some of them have different ways to stay active and on track, so share, and listen.

Chapter 6: Changing the Way You Eat

For a person to lose weight and keep it off, a combination of exercise and eating the right kind and amount of food is needed. It's a shame that most people have resorted to extreme or dangerous measures to lose weight, when it is possible to lose weight through changing one's attitude towards food, and changing one's eating habits. And this can be done not by dramatically cutting back on the amount of food that you eat, nor by depriving yourself of the foods you love, but by developing a well-balanced and satisfying relationship with your food. Healthy eating will certainly make you lose weight, and at the same time reduce your risk of illnesses such as diabetes, heart disease, and certain types of cancer, as well as boost energy and improve your mood.

In our eat-and-run, massive portion sized culture, maintaining a healthy weight can be tough—and losing weight can be even tougher. Adding to the difficulty is the number of fad diets and quick fix methods that tempt and confuse us, and ultimately fail. If you've tried and failed to lose weight before, you might believe that it's just too difficult or that diets don't work for you. And in one sense, you may be right: traditional diets don't work, not for long term weight loss anyway.

But there are a lot of small but powerful changes that you can do that add up to lasting weight loss. The key is to create a plan that provides plenty of enjoyable choices, avoiding common dieting pitfalls, and learning how to develop a healthier, more satisfying relationship with food.

By: E. A Wilson

Healthy eating is not about strict nutrition rules, staying unrealistically and unhealthily thin, or depriving yourself of the foods you love. It's about feeling good, having more energy, stabilizing your mood, and keeping yourself as healthy as possible while maintaining an ideal weight that's right for your body.

How do you know if you are at the right weight? One thing that you could do is to calculate your waist to hips ratio. This is a quick and easy method to estimate body composition and proportions. To do this, using a measuring tape, measure the circumference of your hips at the widest part of your buttocks. Then, measure your waist at the smallest circumference of your natural waist. If you're not sure how to do that, place the tape measure just above your belly button.

Once you've got the measurements, divide your waist measurement by your hip measurement, so the result should look something like this:
Waist measurement: 28 inches
Hip measurement: 39 inches
Waist-to-hip ratio: 28 ÷ 39 = 0.71
For women, the ideal ratio should be no more than 0.8, and for men, it's no more than 0.9. For our example here, this person, who happens to be a woman, has a ratio of 0.71 and appears to be within a healthy range.

Another way to see if you're at the right weight (or if you're gaining or losing weight) is to think about how the waist band of your pants feel. If it's feeling a bit snugger than usual, then you may have to cut back on certain indulgences. Or maybe you'd just like to fit into a pair of pants or a dress that used to fit you like a dream. Again, it's not about being super thin—it's about feeling good in one's own skin. One thing that you could do is to keep a certain article of clothing that makes you look good and feel good whenever you put wear it. Make it your goal to fit into it again. For men, a pair of slacks that have gone tight could be something that could spur you on to lose the excess weight. For women, looking good in a formfitting dress or a pair of nice jeans could be the ultimate reward to weight loss. Focus on these goals, and not the numbers on the scale.

Now let's start on healthy eating. Here are some things that you could do to set yourself up to eating well.

- **Start Slow.**

  Trying to make your diet healthy overnight isn't realistic. Changing everything at once usually leads to cheating or giving up on your diet plan. Make small steps, like adding a salad or soup to your diet once a day. Both are filling and when made with the right ingredients, can be very healthy for you. You can also switch from butter to olive oil or coconut oil when cooking. Instead of deep frying, try sautéing your food in a wok, which uses less oil and keep vegetables crisp while cooking. Cut back on your sugar little by little. It can be hard, especially if you have a sweet tooth. Diabetics should especially take care to lower their glucose intake, as sugar can be found in many forms such as syrups, carb drinks, biscuits, cakes, and creamy desserts.

You could try reducing your sugar intake in simple ways. For instance, if you take your coffee with two teaspoons of sugar, try reducing it by half a teaspoon and stick with it for a week. The following week, reduce it further so you'll be only using one teaspoon of sugar in your coffee. As your small changes become habit, you can continue to add healthy choices to your diet.

- **Simplify**
Instead of being too concerned with counting calories or measuring portion sizes, think of your diet in terms of color, variety and freshness. For example, think back on the last meal that you had today. Did it have vegetables? Did it have at least one kind of fruit? Was there protein and a reasonable amount of carbs? Did you have it with plain water or were you drinking soda as you ate your meal? Did it have too many sweet elements? Thinking about and assessing your diet this way should make it easier to make healthy choices. Focus on finding foods that you love and easy recipes that incorporate a few fresh ingredients. Sometimes, that's really all you need. The fresher the food is, the better it tastes. Anyone who's ever had a fresh tomato, especially one that was picked right off the vine will know how important and how tasty fresh food is. Forego the frozen dinners sold in the supermarket and

head on out to the butcher, the fishmonger, and the farmer's market for a change.

- **Don't strive to be perfect.**
Remember that every change you make to improve your health and your diet matters. You don't have to be perfect and you don't have to eliminate foods you enjoy to have a healthy diet. Think

about your long term goal, which is to feel good, have more energy, and reduce the risk of certain cancers and diseases. Looking and feeling good, having more self confidence, being able to wear nice fitting clothes, attracting members of the opposite sex, or keeping your looks for your husband or boyfriend are all great reasons to lose weight too. Don't let your missteps derail you or discourage you. So you slipped up today and had a big dish of ice cream. That's OK. Tomorrow, you'll make up for it by decreasing your sugar intake and eating a few more helpings of fresh vegetables.

- **Practice moderation.**
Moderation or balance means eating less than what we do now. Specifically, it means eating less of the unhealthy stuff like refined sugars and saturated fat and more of the healthy fare, like fruits and vegetables. But don't worry, it doesn't mean totally eliminating the foods that you love. For example, if you eat bacon once a week, that could be

considered moderation if you follow it up with a healthy lunch and dinner. It's not moderation if you eat bacon once a week then follow it up with a box of donuts or a pepperoni pizza.

- **Don't ban certain foods**
  When you think of certain foods as off limits, it's only natural to want those foods more, and then feel bad once you give in to the temptation to indulge. If you are drawn to sweet, salty or unhealthy foods, start by reducing food portion sizes and not eating them as often. Let's say you make it a habit to eat a whole bag of chips while watching TV. You can limit your consumption by transferring only a handful to a bowl, and keeping the rest of the chips in a tightly covered jar for another day. The same goes for ice cream. If you make it a habit to go through a pint in one sitting, get a small teacup, fill it with ice cream, and keep the rest at the back of your freezer. Better yet, don't buy it if you know that you will only eat it all upon getting home. Once you're sure that you could control your appetite, you can buy a small cup of ice cream (not a pint!) once or twice a week and eat that. Remember to treat yourself only once or twice a week, not every day, as that defeats the purpose of exercising moderation.

A word about carbohydrates. Most people tend to avoid carbs like the plague, thinking that they'll get fat because of carbs. The truth is, eating carbs won't make you fat— but eating too much will. It's the same with other types of

Boiled Potato- plain		Mashed Potato- with butter and whole milk (1 cup) 210 g		French Fried Potato	
Nutrition Facts		Nutrition Facts		Nutrition Facts	
Potato		Mashed Potato		Potato	
Amount Per 100 grams		Amount Per Serving		Amount Per 100 grams	
Calories 77		Calories 237		Calories 312	
% Daily Value		% Daily Value		% Daily Value	
Total Fat 0.1g	0%	Total Fat 9 g	14%	Total Fat 15g	23%
Saturated Fat 0 g	0%	Saturated Fat 4g	22%	Saturated Fat 2.3 g	11%
Polyunsaturated Fat 0 g		Trans Fat 0g		Polyunsaturated Fat 5 g	
Monounsaturated Fat 0 g		Cholesterol 23 mg	8%	Monounsaturated Fat 6 g	
Cholesterol 0 mg	0%	Sodium 666 mg	28%	Cholesterol 0 mg	0%
Sodium 4 mg	0%	Total Carbohydrate 35g	12%	Sodium 210 mg	8%
Potassium 379 mg	10%	Dietary Fiber 3g	13%	Potassium 579 mg	16%
Total Carbohydrate 20 g	6%	Sugars 3g		Total Carbohydrate 41 g	13%
Dietary Fiber 1.8 g	7%	Protein 4g		Dietary Fiber 3.8 g	15%
Sugar 0.9 g				Sugar 0.3 g	
Protein 1.9 g	3%			Protein 3.4 g	6%
Vitamin A 0% Vitamin C 21%		Vitamin A 5% Vitamin C 21%		Vitamin A 0% Vitamin C 7%	
Calcium 0% Iron 1%		Calcium 5% Iron 3%		Calcium 1% Iron 4%	
Vitamin D 0% Vitamin B6 15%				Vitamin D 0% Vitamin B6 20%	
Vitamin... 0% Magnesium 5%				Vitamin... 0% Magnesium 8%	

food: if you eat too much of one thing, it will definitely make you fat, especially if it contains refined sugars such as rice, pasta and spaghetti. Choose healthy carbs and fiber sources, like whole grains, for long lasting energy. They're delicious and satisfying, and are loaded with phytochemicals and antioxidants which help to protect against heart disease, certain cancers and diabetes.

Potatoes are not refined carbs, they are mostly starch. They are high in vitamin C and potassium, and they can only be fattening depending on how you cook them. Let's look at the nutritional value of potatoes prepared in different ways: boiled, mashed, and French fried.

* Per cent values are based on a 2,000 calorie diet. Your daily values are based may be higher or lower depending on your calorie needs.

So far, the dish that has the most calories and fat is the French fried potatoes. The boiled potato has the lowest calories, but it can be quite boring to eat a plain boiled potato every single time. Your best bet would be to have the mashed potato, but to make it healthier, substitute the milk and butter with olive oil and flavor it with garlic and herbs. You'll get the flavor without the unwanted calories and fats.

- **Have smaller portions**

  It's alarming how serving sizes have ballooned recently, particularly in restaurants. Even convenience stores are jumping on the supersized food bandwagon, with sodas available by the bucket. When dining out, choose an appetizer instead of an entrée. You could also split a dish with a friend. Most of all, never agree to supersize anything. When you're at home, use smaller plates. Think about serving sizes in realistic terms, and start small. If you don't feel satisfied at the end of the meal, try adding more fresh vegetables or having fruits for dessert. Use visual cues to help you remember your portion sizes. For example, your protein such as chicken, meat or fish should be about the size of a deck of cards. A slice of bread should be the size of a CD case, and half a cup of mashed potato or rice or pasta is about the size of a traditional light bulb.

- **Focus on eating.**

  Eat together as a family in the dining room, with absolutely no distractions if possible. That means no TV in the dining room, and turning off all cell phones. Eating in front of the TV or computer often leads to mindless overeating. Take time to chew your food and enjoy mealtimes. Make sure to chew your food slowly, and savor each bite. We tend to rush through our meals, forgetting to actually taste the flavors and the textures of our food. When eating at the office, resist eating your meals on your desk, because eating becomes an afterthought, as if nourishing our bodies is not a priority. If you have a pantry, eat your lunch there together with your co-workers. Or if you don't have a pantry and it's a nice day outside, step out, find a nice park or a place where you can eat your lunch, and enjoy your food and the view.

Sometimes, family and friends may have the best intentions of feeding us, only it causes us to pack on the pounds due to the endless buffets and numerous helpings plopped on our plates by well-meaning people. If this is the case, let them know about your goal to lose weight as you're concerned about your health. A lot of people react positively to this rather than if you said that you really want to lose weight to improve your looks (though if this is your real reason, there's no need to let them know about it!) Tell them that you're concerned about your sugar and fat intake, and they'll be more supportive, and it will give them a reason to back off from pressuring you to eat more.

- **Don't forget to eat breakfast**

  Most people think that skipping a meal can help them lose weight, and often, it is breakfast that people tend to forget about eating. A healthy breakfast can jumpstart your metabolism, and eating small, healthy meals throughout the day keeps your energy up and your metabolism going.

- **Listen to your body**

  Before you reach for another helping of food, ask yourself first if you are really hungry. Have a glass of water first before having another bite. If you do feel hungry, then feel free to get more food. During a meal, stop eating before you feel full. It takes a few minutes for your brain to tell your body that it has had enough food, so eat slowly.

- **Avoid eating at night**

  Try to eat dinner earlier in the day. Try having a period of 14 to 16 hours before your next meal, which is breakfast the next day. Studies show that this simple adjustment—eating only when you're most active and giving your digestive system a long break each day—may help to regulate weight. Most after-dinner snacks, like chips or creamy desserts tend to be high in fat and calories, so they should be avoided. Don't load up on sugar or comfort food during dinner. Also, allow a minimum of 4 hours after eating your last meal of the day before going to bed.

- **Load up on colorful vegetables and fruits**

  Fruits and veggies are the foundation of a healthy diet, just like what your mom used to tell you. They are low in calories and full of nutrients, and they're packed with vitamins and minerals, antioxidants and fiber. And while advertisements abound for supplements promising to deliver the nutritional benefits of fruits and vegetables in pill or powder form, to tell you the truth, it's just not the same. A daily regimen of nutritional supplements is not going to have the same impact as eating right. Try to eat a rainbow of fruits and vegetables every day and with every meal—the brighter the color, the better for you. Aim for a minimum of five portions daily.

Chapter 7: Adjusting One's Attitude To Achieve Weight Loss

Your attitude will play a huge factor whether or not you'll be successful at changing your eating habits, losing weight and keeping it off, and improving your health.

If you think you were born to be fat and there's nothing that can change that, then you should know that a USDA study found that women who think that their genes regulate their waist size are more likely to be heavy. Your genes do have an impact on your weight. But it's the everyday choices you make that determine how large you become.

Start thinking that the food and lifestyle choices you make today will determine your shape. Put yourself in situations where you are likely to be successful in choosing healthful foods until you build a history of success. You could do this in simple ways, such as avoiding the junk food and candy aisles at the grocery and steering your cart towards fresh produce and more healthful choices. Or take a different route to work because every time you pass by the cupcake shop, you can't resist popping in to buy a cupcake or two. Remember, small things like these can add up to weight loss.

Do you hear yourself saying, "There's no way I'll ever lose this weight!" If you might have said it a lot of times, you might be setting your expectations too high. If you think you need to get back to your high school weight, no wonder you're feeling overwhelmed! Truth is, even if you lose only five to eight pounds during the first month, there's already a big difference in the way you'll feel. Somehow, you feel lighter and more energetic. Your clothes fit a lot looser, and that itself can be a pleasant change. Don't step on a scale and use that as a gauge for weight loss—it's much better to see if you're losing weight by checking the way your clothes fit. Learn how to set reasonable but challenging goals that will lead to long term weight loss success.

If you're baffled that you're not eating much yet you seem to be unable to lose weight, remember that you have to take into account every morsel of food and drink that passes your lips. Even just a small slice of pizza eaten every day can affect your weight. Work with the facts and choose healthy foods with no refined sugars or unhealthy carbs.

Remember that slow and steady wins the race. Aim to lose one to two pounds a week to ensure healthy weight loss. Losing weight too fast can take a toll on your mind and body, and this can make you feel sluggish and sick. When you drop a lot of weight quickly, you're actually losing mostly water and muscle, rather than fat. This is why people who take weight loss pills tend to look haggard or drained, as opposed to the healthy, glowing look that comes with doing the right way to achieve weight loss.

Think of weight loss as a lifestyle change, not a short term diet. Permanent weight loss is not something that a quick fix diet can achieve. It's a lifestyle change, a commitment to improve your health for life. True, various fad diets can help jumpstart weight loss, but permanent changes in your lifestyle and food choices will work even better.

Soup Recipes

Soup is a quick, hot meal that offers plenty of benefits. You can pop in some ingredients into a crock pot to cook slowly, and it will be ready by the time you get home from work. You can even freeze individual portions and heat them up before eating. You can also prepare a quick soup in just under 20 minutes. It's easy, relatively inexpensive to make, and filled with fiber, nutrients, vitamins, and can make you feel good when you're feeling under the weather. Eating a bowl of soup as an appetizer or as a quick meal by itself is also a great way to cut down on the calories. As an appetizer, it leaves you feeling full before your main course, so you eat less of the heavier foods. If you choose to make soup as your main meal, you can always make it more appealing by adding your favorite bread or some low sodium crackers on the side.

Whether you're eating a bowl for lunch or dinner, the more homemade soup you consume instead of other foods, the less calories you will consume, which will lead to weight loss. For those who want a more intense regime, a vegetable soup can replace two meals a day for five to seven days without any side effects. Although much of the weight loss will be fluid, sometimes all we need to feel leaner and healthier is a flatter stomach and a pound or two less on the scales.

However, not all soups can be good for your health. Cream-based soups such as chowders can be laden with calories. If you choose to make, say, a clam chowder, substitute milk for cream to cut down on the richness. Cook soups that are more brothy than creamy, as a lot of broth-based soups include plenty of vegetables, and the flavor comes from the veggies and the protein.

Vegetable Minestrone Soup

This very healthy minestrone is bound to fill you up, and is filled with seven kinds of vegetables.

Yield: 6-8 servings

Ingredients:

2 tablespoons olive oil

1 medium yellow onion

2 teaspoons minced garlic

2 teaspoons fresh oregano, chopped

2 medium zucchini, chopped (or 2 cups of broccoli florets, if you can't find it)

2 medium yellow squash, chopped

2 medium carrots, chopped

One 15-ounce can whole kernel sweet white corn, drained

6 tomatoes, chopped and divided into 3 cups and 1 cup

Three 14-ounce cans low sodium chicken broth

½ cup uncooked ditalini pasta (or dried elbow macaroni pasta)

One 15-ounce can or white beans, rinsed and drained

Two handfuls of baby spinach

¾ teaspoon kosher or sea salt

¼ teaspoon freshly ground black pepper

1 cup grated parmesan cheese

Instructions:

- Heat oil in a saucepan or soup pot over medium heat.
- Add the onion to the pan. Saute' for 3 minutes until softened, stirring frequently.
- Add the oregano and garlic, saute' for 1 minute, stirring frequently.

- Stir in the squash, zucchini or broccoli, carrots and corn. Saute' for 5 minutes until vegetables are tender, stirring occasionally.
- While the vegetables are cooking, place 3 cups chopped tomatoes and 1 can of broth in a blender. Blend until smooth.
- Add the tomato mixture to the pot. Stir in the remaining tomatoes and the rest of the broth. Bring to a boil. Reduce the heat and simmer for 20 minutes.
- Add pasta and beans to cook. Cook for 10 minutes until pasta is tender. Stir occasionally.
- Remove from heat. Stir in the spinach, salt and pepper.

Ladle soup into bowls and top each bowl with 2 tablespoons of grated cheese.

Tilapia Corn Chowder

This soup is a great alternative to clam chowder. Strewn with fresh, sweet corn and tilapia, it's a fine meal by itself, just add a green salad and some oyster crackers to complete it.

Yield: 6 servings
Ingredients:
2 ounces bacon
1 teaspoon vegetable oil
1 stalk celery, diced
1 leek, white part only, halved lengthwise, rinsed and sliced thinly
½ teaspoon salt
½ teaspoon pepper
4 cups reduced sodium chicken broth
8 Yukon Gold or russet potatoes, diced
2 cups fresh corn kernels
1 ½ pound or 0.6 kg. tilapia fillets
1 teaspoon finely chopped fresh thyme
1 cup milk
2 teaspoons lemon juice
2 chopped fresh chives

Instructions:
- Chop bacon and cook in a large sauce pan or Dutch oven over medium heat until crispy. Drain on paper towels and set aside.
- Add oil to the pan. Add celery, leek, salt and pepper and cook until the vegetables start to soften.

- Add the broth, potatoes and corn. Bring to a gentle simmer. Cook until the potatoes are just tender and the corn is cooked through.
- Stir in tilapia and thyme. Return to a gentle simmer. Cook until the tilapia is cooked through. Remove from heat.

Stir in the milk, lemon juice, and the reserved bacon. Garnish with chives.

Tomato and Orzo Soup

This soup has a rich and creamy texture, though it doesn't have even a drop of cream in it! It's satisfying, and is a great soup to have especially on cold nights.

Yield: Serves 6
Ingredients:
½ onion, chopped
1 tablespoon olive oil
2 cloves garlic, minced
Three 15-ounce cans diced tomato
½ cup Greek yoghurt
2 bay leaves
One 15-ounce can or vegetable broth
1 teaspoon brown sugar
¼ cup chopped fresh basil
A dash of crushed red pepper flakes
salt and ground pepper to taste
1 cup cooked orzo pasta

Instructions:
- In a large pot, heat the olive oil over medium heat. Add the onion and garlic and cook until tender. Stir in the bay leaves.
- Add the tomatoes and vegetable broth.
- Stir in the brown sugar and fresh basil. Season with red pepper flakes, salt and pepper to taste. Simmer over low heat for 15 minutes.

- Remove the bay leaves from the pot. Use an immersion blender to blend the soup. You could also use a blender to do this, then return the soup to the pot.
- Stir in the Greek yoghurt until well combined.

Add the orzo pasta. Stir and serve warm.

Potato Cauliflower Soup

A lot of traditional potato soups call for ham or bacon. This is a healthier version that is packed with Vitamin B nutrients from fiber-rich cauliflower. For an even healthier twist, try making this soup using sweet potatoes.

Yield: Serves 4
Ingredients:
Croutons:
1 teaspoon ground cumin
1 teaspoon olive oil
1 cup cubed French bread

Soup:
2 teaspoons olive oil
1/3 cup finely chopped shallots (or 1/3 cup chopped onion with 1 minced garlic)
1/3 cup finely chopped celery
2 ½ cups sliced cauliflower
¾ pound or 0.3 kg of sliced and peeled Yukon gold or russet potatoes
Two 14 ounce cans low sodium chicken broth
½ teaspoon salt
¼ teaspoon ground black pepper
1 teaspoon lemon juice
2 teaspoons chopped chives

Instructions:
To make the croutons:
- Preheat oven to 350 degrees

- Combine cumin and 1 teaspoon olive oil in bowl. Add the bread cubes, then toss to coat.
- Spread bread cubes on a baking sheet and bake at 350 degrees for 10 minutes or until golden.
- Cool croutons slightly and set aside.

To make the soup:
- Heat 2 teaspoons oil in a large saucepan over medium heat.
- Add the shallots or onion with garlic and the celery. Cover and cook for 2 minutes.
- Stir in the cauliflower, potato, chicken broth, salt and pepper. Bring to a boil.
- Reduce the heat, cover, and simmer for 15 to 20 minutes or until vegetables are tender.
- Add the lemon juice.
- Place the vegetable soup in batches in a food processor or blender and process or blend until smooth.
- Divide the soup evenly among 4 bowls

Serve with croutons and garnish with the chopped chives.

Cream of Asparagus and Leek Soup

This is a delicious soup that evokes the flavors of spring and is so good for you.
It's low in calories, yet big on flavor.

Yield: 4 servings
Ingredients:
2 leeks, cut into thin slices (make sure to only use the white or yellow part of the leek)
1 medium onion, diced
4 stalks of celery, diced
2 tablespoons olive oil
4 medium potatoes, peeled and diced
3 cups of chicken stock or broth
1 ½ teaspoons salt
1 teaspoon onion powder
1 teaspoon chopped parsley
¼ teaspoon garlic powder
1/8 teaspoon thyme
a pinch of dried sage
20 spears of asparagus, with the tough ends removed and sliced into half inch pieces.
1 cup of almond milk

Instructions:
- In a large saucepan, saute' leeks, onions, and celery in oil over low heat for 5 minutes.
- Turn heat on high and add the potatoes to the pan along with two cups of the chicken stock or broth and the seasonings.

- Cover the saucepan and bring to a boil. When the soup comes to a boil, reduce heat to medium and cook until potatoes are tender, but not soft (about 4-5 minutes).
- Remove 2 cups of the soup mixture from the saucepan and pour into a blender and set aside.
- Stir the remaining cup of chicken stock or broth and asparagus pieces into the remaining soup in the saucepan. Cook uncovered at a low boil for 5 minutes.
- While the soup is cooking, add the almond milk to the mixture in the blender, and blend until smooth.
- Stir in the blender mixture into the soup in the saucepan. Cook until thoroughly heate

Salad Recipes

Salads composed even from few ingredients have a lot of health benefits, especially if most of the elements are made up of fruits or vegetables. Incorporating the occasional salad into your diet can be very beneficial for you.

If you're aiming for weight loss, a salad can be one of the most satisfying ways to consume a few calories. A nice, hearty serving will have about the same calories as one slice of bread, won't cause a blood sugar spike, will help prevent obesity and its health complications, and is a lot more filling. It's filling because vegetables contain a lot of water, and also because salads are high in fiber, which makes you feel full. Salads also contribute to heart health because anti-oxidants like Vitamin C and E are in most salad ingredients such as broccoli, strawberries, sunflower seeds and spinach. Antioxidants may also play a role in preventing cancer.

Though it is a given that salad is a healthy food, it won't help you slim down if the veggies are weighed down by a pound of cheese. The same goes for salads with a pint of croutons, swimming in little pools of creamy dressing, and loaded with calorie-dense dried fruit and full of high-fat nuts. On the other hand, you could be missing out on the health benefits of salad if you only prepare one that's mostly all lettuce leaves with a smidgen of vinaigrette. Here are some tips on how to make a healthful salad.

- Pile on the vegetables. Choose a variety of colors to get the most health benefits, such as combining red bell

- peppers and broccoli with carrots, sugar snap peas, cucumbers and red onions. Stick with raw or lightly steamed vegetables only and steer clear of ones that are fried.
- Add some protein. When you add protein to your salad, it becomes a meal by itself. If you're adding animal protein, select the lean kind such as skinless chicken, turkey breast, light tuna, wild salmon, or lean sirloin steak. Vegetarians can get protein from cubed tofu or chickpeas, kidney beans, pinto beans, or other legumes.
- Choose one extra ingredient. Now some of these extras are packed with nutrients, but they're also rich in calories and fat—thus, they should be added sparingly. Choose from one of the following: grated cheddar, parmesan, goat, Swiss, or feta cheese; chopped nuts such as walnuts, pecans, or almonds; avocado, olives, croutons, and dried fruit. Cheese should be no more than 2 teaspoons per serving, chopped nuts should not exceed more than one tablespoon. One ounce of avocado is just right, as well as ¼ cup of croutons, and 2 tablespoons of dried fruit will suffice.

Dress salads lightly. Limit your dressing to one and a half tablespoons for an entrée salad and one teaspoon for a side salad. Whenever possible, choose low calorie or low fat options. Better yet, make your own salad dressing instead of using those that come from a jar or bottle—it's healthier and has no additives or preservatives.

Grilled Chicken Pasta Salad

This is a twist on the classic Caesar salad. The pasta and grilled chicken makes this a complete meal that everyone will surely love, and instead of Ceasar dressing, homemade Dijon vinaigrette brightens the flavors of the greens. .
Yield: Makes 6 servings

Ingredients
For the dressing:
2 cloves of garlic, minced
½ teaspoon Dijon mustard
1 tablespoon or more of lemon juice, to taste
3 tablespoons extra virgin olive oil
salt and black pepper, to taste
For the salad:
3 cups grilled chicken, cut into bite size pieces
6 ounces penne pasta, cooked and cooled
4 cups Romaine lettuce, cut into small pieces
1 cucumber, diced
¼ cup fresh basil, thinly sliced
¼ cup green onions, thinly sliced
2 cups halved cherry tomatoes

Instructions:
- To make the dressing, place the garlic, mustard, lemon juice, and oil in a small jar. Season with salt and pepper.
- Shake the jar vigorously to combine. Adjust seasonings if necessary.
- In a bowl, toss all the salad ingredients with the dressing.
Serve immediately.

By: E. A Wilson

Kale Salad with Cranberry Vinaigrette

Kale is a wonderful leafy vegetable, and is currently very trendy for those who are into healthy eating. The flavor of kale is greatly enhanced when paired with a sweet and savory vinaigrette.
Yield: 2-4 servings

Ingredients:
3 tbsp olive oil
1 shallot or 1 small red onion, peeled and thinly sliced
3 cloves of garlic, coarsely chopped
1 cup dried cranberries
2 tbsp. red wine vinegar or cider vinegar
juice and zest of half a lemon
1/8 teaspoon salt
1/8 teaspoon ground black pepper
1 bunch of kale, thinly sliced
¼ cup almonds

Instructions:
- In a small saucepan, saute' the garlic and shallot in olive oil.
- Whisk in the lemon juice, vinegar, salt and pepper.
- Add the cranberries to the pan. Cook for about 1 minute, then remove from heat.
- In a bowl, place the kale and toss with the warm dressing.
Add the almonds, toss and serve.

Broccoli Salad

This is a healthy, hearty salad loaded with broccoli, plump grapes and crunchy pecans tossed in a Greek yoghurt dressing for that extra zing.

Yield: 6 servings
Ingredients:
For the dressing:
½ cup plain Greek yoghurt
½ cup mayonnaise
1/3 cup red wine vinegar
1 tablespoon sugar
½ teaspoon dried thyme
kosher salt and freshly ground pepper to taste

For the salad:
6 slices of lean bacon, diced
8 ounces bowtie or penne pasta
1 head broccoli, cut into florets and finely chopped
2 cups seedless red grapes, halved
1/3 cup red onion, diced
¼ cup chopped pecans

Instructions:
- To make the dressing, whisk together the yoghurt, mayonnaise, vinegar, thyme, salt and pepper in a small bowl. Set it aside.
- In a large pot of boiling salted water, cook pasta according to package instructions. Drain well.

- In a large skillet over medium heat, cook the bacon until crispy. Transfer to a plate lined with a paper towel.
- In a large bowl, combine pasta, bacon, broccoli, grapes, red onion, pecan and dressing. Serve immediately.

Fresh Fruit Salad with Creamy Yoghurt Dressing

A fruit salad is great as a palate cleanser, a snack, or as a healthy end to a delicious meal. Keep calories low by using Greek yoghurt instead of heavy cream.

Yield: 8 servings
Ingredients:
2 cups of fresh strawberries
2 peaches, sliced
2 bananas, sliced
2 cups of red or green grapes
8 ounces plain or Greek yoghurt
2 teaspoons lemon juice
1 teaspoon brown sugar
½ teaspoon vanilla extract
3 tablespoons lime juice

Instructions:
- In a small bowl, mix together the yoghurt, lemon juice, sugar, and vanilla. Set aside.
- Mix all the fruits in a large bowl. Mix in the lime juice to keep the fruit from going brown.
- Serve the yoghurt mix separately. It can be used as a dip for the fruit, or it can be mixed in with the fruit to make the salad.

Alternative fruits that you could use are blueberries, kiwis, cantaloupe, and pineapple. Use whatever is in season.

Healthy Chef Salad

Most chef salads that you see in restaurants are laden with ingredients which can do more harm than good. We put a healthy spin on this classic salad by using chicken breast instead of bacon, and a homemade ranch dressing instead of one from a bottle.

Yield: 8 servings
Ingredients:
For the dressing:
½ cup buttermilk (or half a teaspoon of lemon juice stirred in half a cup of milk if you don't have it)
½ cup Greek yoghurt
¼ cup dill, finely chopped
¼ teaspoon freshly ground pepper
¼ teaspoon salt
¼ teaspoon garlic powder

For the salad:
½ head iceberg lettuce, roughly chopped
½ cucumber, sliced into rounds
2 medium tomatoes, roughly chopped
2 eggs, boiled and sliced
8 ounces cooked chicken breast, chopped
¼ cup grated parmesan cheese

Instructions:
- For the salad dressing, combine all ingredients and in a jar and shake vigorously. Refrigerate for at least 30 minutes for best results.

Toss the salad ingredients in a large bowl and top with the dressing.

Stew Recipes

Winter or rainy season brings cravings for comfort food—heavy casseroles and rich stews that make us feel warm from the inside-out against the cold weather.

The problem is, most comfort food—like stew, for instance—doesn't score high marks in the healthy column. In fact, a lot of stew recipes are packed with calories, fat, and salt.

However, it is possible to eat hearty and healthy. One thing that you could do is to watch your portion size before tinkering with the recipe. One serving of stew should be about one cup or one small bowl, enough to make you feel satisfied, but not stuffed.

Next, rethink your ingredients. Add more vegetables to boost the nutritional benefits of your stew. If you don't have fresh vegetables on hand, even canned versions will do. Replace some or all of the cream in the recipe with low fat milk. This will give you the creaminess that you need without the added calories.

Consider the cuts of meat that you put in your stew. Tough cuts of meat that lend themselves to stews tend to be fatty, so you need to trim them well for healthy results. Experiment with other sources of protein such as fish or tofu to add heft to your stew.

By: E. A Wilson

For a good stew, cut all vegetables and meat into roughly equal sizes so that they'll cook evenly. Make sure to cook it on low fire and let it simmer, not boil. You could also use a slow cooker to make it—all you need to do is put all the ingredients in, set the timer, and head out the door. When you get home, your kitchen will be filled with the wonderful aroma of home-cooked goodness.

Healthy Beef Stew

This stew is hearty and especially good for folks on restricted diets, because most of its flavor comes from herbs and spices.
Yield: 6 servings

Ingredients:
6 tablespoons all purpose flour
1 teaspoon paprika
¼ teaspoon pepper
1 ½ lbs. or 0.6 kg beef stew meat, cut into 1-inch cubes
1 tablespoon canola oil
2 cups water
3 tablespoons tomato paste
1 beef bouillon cube
2 tablespoons dried basil
1 teaspoon dried thyme
1 teaspoon garlic powder
2 bay leaves
3 cups peeled potatoes, cubed
3 cups peeled onions, cut into quarters
2 cups sliced carrots
2 tablespoons minced fresh parsley
¼ teaspoon salt
¼ cup cold water

Instructions:
- In a large resealable plastic bag, combine 4 tablespoons flour, paprika and pepper. Add beef a few pieces at a time, and shake to coat.

- In a Dutch oven, brown beef in oil over medium heat. Add the water, tomato paste, beef bouillon, 1 ½ teaspoons basil, ¾ teaspoon thyme, ¾ teaspoon garlic powder, and bay leaves. Bring to a boil, then reduce heat. Cover and simmer for 1 ½ hours.
- Add the potatoes, carrots, and onions. Cover and simmer for 30 minutes.
- Discard the bay leaves. In a small bowl, combine the parsley, salt, and the remaining flour, basil, thyme, and garlic powder. Add the cold water. Stir until smooth.
- Stir the mixture into the stew. Bring to a boil, then stir until thickened.

Chicken and Mushroom Stew

This stew tastes exactly like chicken pot pie, minus the crust. You can use leftover chicken, or buy a rotisserie chicken to cut down on the prep time.
Yield: 4 servings

Ingredients:
2 tablespoons olive oil
½ large white onion, chopped
1 ½ cups chopped celery, including the leaves
2 carrots, chopped
1 cup button mushrooms, sliced
2 cloves garlic, minced
2 potatoes, diced
2 bay leaves
a pinch of dried rosemary and thyme
3 cups cooked chicken, shredded
4 cups chicken broth
2 tablespoons butter
2 tablespoons flour
2 cups of low fat milk
2 tablespoons cornstarch mixed with ¼ cup of water (to thicken the stew)

Instructions:
- In a soup pot, heat 2 tablespoons olive oil and add the chopped onion, celery, carrots, mushrooms, garlic, potatoes, and spices.

- Add the chicken broth to the pot. Bring to a boil, then lower the heat and simmer gently until the vegetables are soft.
- In another small pot, melt the butter. Add the flour and whisk together until combined. Lower the heat and make sure to not let the mixture turn brown. Slowly add the milk, making sure to stir constantly so lumps don't form. When the mixture is thick, add this to the stew and stir well.
- Let the stew simmer for 5 minutes. Season with salt and pepper.
- Add the cornstarch mixed with water if the soup needs further thickening. Bring the pot to a gentle boil and stir. Then lower the heat and simmer for 5 minutes.Garnish with chopped parsley, chives, or jalapeños.

Tilapia Stew

This simple stew is best served with a simple green salad on the side or a piece of crusty bread. You can use any white fish fillet if you can't find tilapia, such as flathead or cream dory.
Yield: 4 servings

Ingredients:
3 tablespoons canola oil
2 onions, peeled and chopped
1 large bulb fennel, trimmed and sliced crosswise, green fronds reserved
1 ½ cups tomato puree or tomato pasta sauce
a pinch of saffron threads
1 pound or 0.6 kg of tilapia, flathead, or cream dory fillets, chopped
1 ½ cups water

Instructions:
- Heat some oil in a large pot. Add the onions and cook over low heat, covered for about 5 minutes.
- Add the fennel and continue to cook then cover it. Stir occasionally for about 10 to 15 minutes or until the onion and fennel are soft but not browned.
- Add the tomato puree or sauce, 1 ½ cups water and saffron. Bring to a simmer.
- Add the fish and cook for about 1 minute. Then remove from the heat and serve while still hot.

White Bean Stew With Kale

Kale adds an earthy flavor to this vegetable stew that takes less than 30 minutes to prepare.
Yield: 4 servings

Ingredients:
4 slices bacon, cut into ½ inch pieces
1 small onion, chopped
2 cans (15 ounce each) cannellini beans, drained and rinsed
1 teaspoon fresh rosemary, chopped
1 cup chicken broth
1 bunch kale, rinsed, trimmed and cut into 1 inch pieces
1/8 teaspoon salt
1/8 teaspoon pepper

Instructions:
- Cook bacon over medium heat until crisp. Place on a plate lined with a paper towel. Set aside.
- In a pot, add the onion and cook for 5 minutes or until softened. Stir in the beans and rosemary and cook for 1 minute.
- Add broth to the pot and bring to a simmer.
- Stir kale into the pot and cover. Cook for 5 minutes. Remove cover and stir until kale is wilted. Stir in the reserved bacon, salt and pepper. Serve immediately.

Lamb and Vegetable Soup

This is a low-fat soup that combines lamb and vegetables for a quick and delicious meal.
Yield: 5 servings

Ingredients:
1 pound or 0.6 kg of lean boneless lamb, cut into ¾ cubes
1 tablespoon cooking oil
One 14 ounce can of beef broth
1 cup beef broth
1 teaspoon dried thyme
2 cloves garlic, minced
1 bay leaf
2 cups butternut squash, peeled and cubed
1 cup sweet potato, peeled and chopped
1 cup sliced celery
1 medium onion, cut into thin wedges
½ cup plain yoghurt or low fat sour cream
3 tablespoons all purpose flour

Instructions:
- In a large saucepan, brown the meat, half at a time, in hot oil. Drain the fat.
- Return the meat to the pan. Stir in the broth, dried thyme, garlic and bay leaf. Bring to a boil, then reduce the heat. Cover and let it simmer for 20 minutes.
- Stir in squash, sweet potato, celery and onion. Bring to a boil, then reduce heat. Cover the pan and let it simmer for 30 minutes or until the meat and vegetables are tender. Discard bay leaf.

- In a small bowl, combine yoghurt and flour. Stir ½ cup of the hot liquid from the stew into the yoghurt mixture. Add the yoghurt mixture to the pan. Cook and stir until thickened and bubbly. Season to taste with salt and pepper.

Snacks Recipes

There seems to be a big divide between those who think that snacking is a good thing and those who think that snacking is bad. To some, snacking means "eating when you're not hungry" or "eating snack foods". But when it's done right, snacking can be a healthy habit that may help you manage your weight and balance your diet.

Smart snacking may help prevent you from overeating at meal times. Most of us get hungry about every 3 to 4 hours after eating. So if there's a long stretch between meals, you're likely to get hungry, which is why a snack would be appropriate. If you resist the urge to snack and hold off until meal time, you'll end up overeating at your next meal.

Smart snacking can also help you work in more healthy foods into your day. The more often you eat, the easier it will be to work in your recommended dietary allowance of healthy foods like vegetables, fruits, and calcium-rich dairy products.

A healthy snack can also help you reduce your overall calorie intake for the day. It can also help you maintain your physical and mental energy. When you eat regular meals and snacks, it can help keep your blood sugar more stable throughout the day.

By: E. A Wilson

That being said, there are indeed many benefits of snacking during the day, but as with all things, too much of a good thing can become a bad thing. As always, watch your portions. Think of food as fuel to get you through the day, so eat snacks to feel good, not to feel stuffed. Also, be selective about the types of snacks that you eat. Snack foods such as chips, fried things, sweet pastries and the like are laden with calories and may make you feel worse. But foods like fruits, vegetables, nuts, low fat milk, whole grains and legumes are satisfying and are packed with nutrients, fiber, and protein that your body needs, and they guard against sugar highs or lows, so you are less likely to succumb to your sweet tooth—or whatever your dietary weakness may be.

Tomato Salsa with Cucumber Dippers

Replace the store-bought chips and dip with this healthy and refreshing tomato salsa with cucumber dippers. It's delicious served after it's made, but the flavors meld nicely after a day in the refrigerator.

Yield: 6 servings

Ingredients:
3 cups tomatoes, finely chopped
½ cup white onion, finely chopped
½ cup finely chopped cilantro
1 small jalapeño, seeded and minced
2 tablespoons fresh lime juice
salt and freshly ground pepper to taste
1 large seedless cucumber, sliced into ¼ inch thick rounds

Instructions:
- In a bowl, toss the tomatoes with the onion, cilantro, jalapeño, and lime juice and season with salt and pepper.

Serve the salsa with the cucumber chips for dipping.

Low Fat Banana Blueberry Muffins

These muffins contain no butter or oil, and are made with whole wheat flour. The addition of Greek yoghurt, blueberries, and bananas make this a yummy yet healthy treat.
Yield: 15 muffins

Ingredients:
2 ½ cups whole wheat flour
1 teaspoon baking soda
¼ teaspoon salt
½ teaspoon cinnamon
¼ cup honey
½ cup brown sugar, loosely packed
1 cup very ripe banana, mashed
¼ cup nonfat Greek yoghurt
1 large egg, beaten
¾ cup almond milk (you can also use soymilk if you want)
1 ¼ cup fresh or unthawed frozen blueberries

Instructions:
- Preheat oven to 325 degrees. Spray muffin tins with nonstick spray and set aside.In a large bowl, gently mix the flour, baking soda, salt, and cinnamon together until well combined. Set aside.
- In a separate bowl, mix the honey and brown sugar together until smooth and free of lumps. Add the mashed banana, yoghurt, and beaten egg. Slowly pour the wet ingredients into the dry ingredients. Gently fold it all together.Add the milk slowly continue to gently mix the

batter. Fold in the blueberries. Do not overmix as this will result to dry, tough muffins.

- Divide the batter between 15 muffin tins. Fill each tin all the way to the pan. Bake for 17-18 minutes until very lightly browned at the edges.
- Cool the muffins before serving.

Turkey and Tomato Sandwich

A creamy spread with parmesan and basil flavors a turkey and tomato sandwich for a savory snack.

Yield: 4 servings

Ingredients:

3 tablespoons reduced fat mayonnaise
2 tablespoons shredded Parmesan cheese
2 tablespoons plain nonfat yoghurt
2 tablespoons chopped fresh basil
1 teaspoon lemon juice
freshly ground pepper to taste
8 slices whole wheat bread
8 ounces thinly sliced turkey breast
8 tomato slices

Instructions:

- In a bowl, combine mayonnaise, yoghurt, Parmesan, basil, lemon juice, and pepper.
- Spread about 2 tablespoons of the mixture on each slice of bread. Divide the turkey and tomato slices among 4 slices of bread, then top with the remaining bread.

Toast the sandwiches in an oven toaster for about 4 minutes on medium heat.

Mixed Berry Yoghurt Parfait

Craving for something cold, sweet and creamy? Before you reach for that tub of ice cream, try making this berry yoghurt parfait. It's naturally sweet, creamy, and so good for you.
Yield: 1 serving

Ingredients:
½ cup blueberries
½ cup strawberries
½ cup raspberries
2 teaspoons of brown sugar
1 cup low fat yoghurt or Greek yoghurt
½ cup low fat granola
1 tablespoon of chopped walnuts

Instructions:
- Mix the berries and sugar. Stir well and set aside.
- Using a spoon, scoop up half of the berry mixture and place in a glass.
- Top the fruit with half of the yoghurt, then half of the granola.
- Continue layering with the remaining fruit, yoghurt, and granola.

Sprinkle with walnuts on top.

White Bean and Artichoke Dip

Eating plain vegetables can get pretty boring after a while. But serve them up with this delicious dip, and you'll see just how good veggies can taste.
Yield: 2 cups of dip

Ingredients:
2 cloves garlic
2 (15 ounce) cans white beans, drained and rinsed
1 (15 ounce) can artichoke hearts, drained
3 tablespoons fresh lemon juice
1 teaspoon red pepper flakes
1 tablespoon chopped rosemary
salt and pepper to taste

Instructions:
- In a food processor, add the garlic, white beans, artichoke hearts, lemon juice, red pepper flakes, and rosemary. Blend until smooth.
- Season with salt and pepper and mix well. Serve with vegetables, bread, or crackers. This dip can also be used as a spread.